THE BEST GUIDE ON HOW TO MAKE YOUR PENIS BIGGER

Detailed Step in Getting the Easy Way of Using Natural Supplements, Exercise and Correct Diet Plans to

Achieve Bigger, Stronger and Thicker penis Legally & Cheap

BY

DOCTOR ELIZA PARKER

copyright@2018

TABLE OF CONTENT

CHAPTER ONE

INTRODUCTION

If you know that you want to be called a proper man that has a big, strong penis that has come to be with the help of a simple guide on natural penis enlargement which has no side effect.

Your penis can be strengthen naturally with just some simple tip and tricks you need to know.

1. THE USE OF NATURAL SUPPLEMENT FOR PENIS ENLARGEMENT

A useful supplement is very important to be taking for you to experience and have a bigger and strong penis. You will have to allow the natural ingredient to perform its function by making the length and girth increase naturally.

There is nothing you can do to make your penis bigger genuinely except you will have to back up your exercise with natural supplement. It is also very safe way because that is when you will observe and see your penis really getting bigger in size.

You cannot rely on exercise alone because it does not give quick and faster result as compare to natural supplements.

You must note that for you to notice or experience a better result in your penis enlargement, the correct brand of natural supplement is what you must buy and take since it has no side effects. Series of studies has been carried out and several changes has been done with natural supplements and therefore making it more useful and reliable

This is the safest and recommended way for penis enlargement since it is supported by several clinical researches.

Vital things to consider in a supplement are the

- It must be a natural a supplement

- It must contain approved ingredient

- It must worth its cost

- It must be easy to use

Some of the ingredients it must contain which are needed for blood flow, libido and size are:

Amino acids, herbs and nutrient.

Get a well recommended natural supplement from a reliable source.

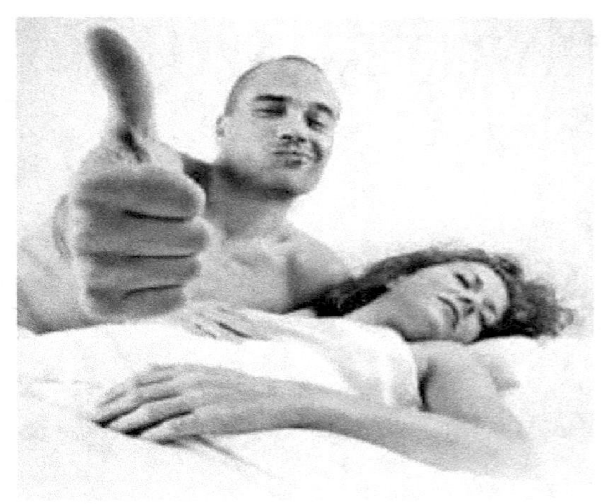

CHAPTER TWO

DO PENIS EXERCISE

Working out every day is what you need to quickly increase your penis effectively. Your body will come up in good shape and a nice self-esteem when you carry out frequent exercise. When your body is good, you will have sex satisfaction and increase penis. Below are several reliable penis exercises that are working very well for men

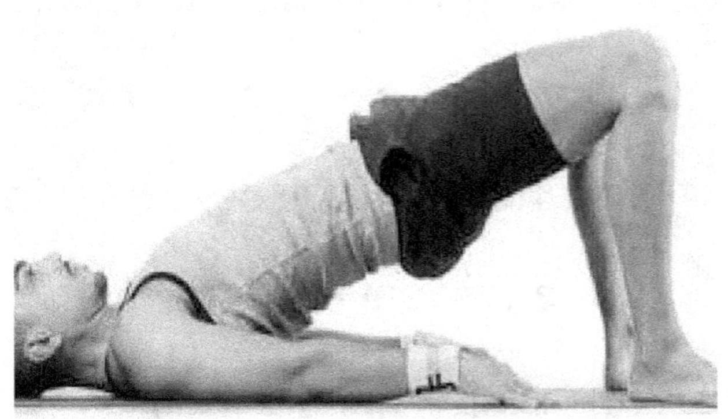

A. WALLY WALLY UP

This penis enlargement exercise is carried out when you retrieve your erectile phase by the act of sitting at the tip of a chair. Get a towel and with it hold the penis head and increase it for duration of three or six seconds. It can be done for up to five several phases.

After this exercise if you feel stronger, you can raise the

resistance with the use of a wet or large towel over the penis head. Before any exercise is carried out, it advised you warm up by getting a warm cloth and water which you will use to squeeze it correctly. Adhering to this exercise guide will make you have large, bigger and stronger penis significantly without side effects caused by medications.

This pennies enlargement exercise should be done regularly and for longer period of time so as to get better results.

B. THE USE OF LUBRICATION

The warming process is what must be done before moving on to this stage of lubrication exercise which is another vital stage in penis enlargement naturally. There a lot of lubricant out there but the suitable must be petroleum or water based lubricant. The lubricant I recommend is oil lubricant which contain

- ✓ Vitamin complexes
- ✓ Botanical extracts
- ✓ Antioxidants

These content moves straight into the tissues

of the penis for quick and targeted results of penis enlargement.

Remember that water lubricant dries out faster so make sure the oil lubricant is what you will use.

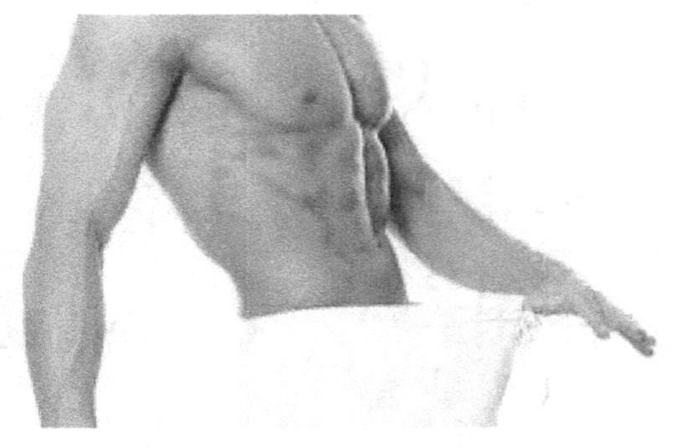

B. USE STRETCHES FOR PENIS

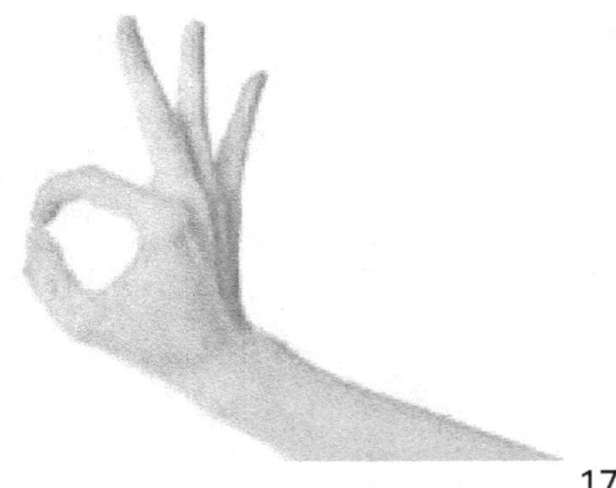

What to do first is to hold firmly your penis which is another enhancement exercise. Place one hand around the head of your penis and place the other hand around the other hand. Since you have hold the penis, stretch it and rotate it towards the left hand side for 25 times to 30 times and then take a rest. Sooner you will massage your penis a little, hold it and rotate it this time to the right hand side for 25 times or 30 times before taking a little break

This exercise should be carried out daily so as to get a speedy results of enlarge and stronger penis. The stretching exercise will be painful when you do not perform the warm up exercise first. Stretching exercise is recognized as one of the accepted fastest penis enlargement exercise but it needs you to be patient enough and making sure it is performed rightly.

If you will not feel any pain without using the warm up exercise or pills, go ahead with the penis stretching

exercise   for   your
enlargement.

D.USE LENGTH EXTENDER

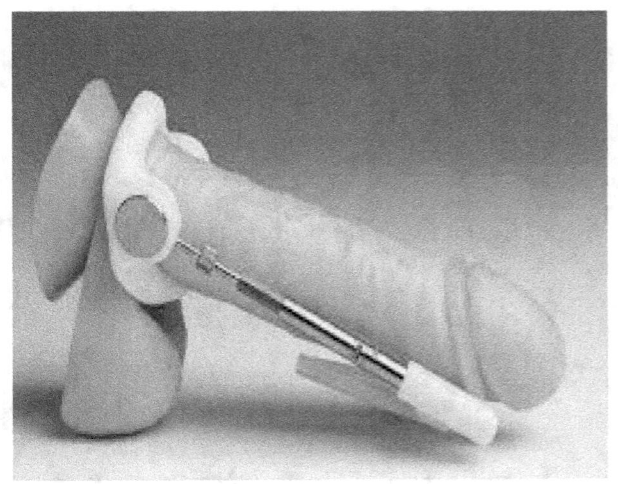

Hold the penis firmly at the head and the other hand is used to make a grip. You can either take a standing or sitting position. The penis head should be held straight for at least 25 seconds. You can now pull the penis and also stretch it. This exercise can be painful when doing it and sooner take a little break and repeat the process for better and quicker enhancement.

This extender is so designed in a way that it gives gentle penis traction. This device is placed around the penis base and also around the head (corona glans) which give full adjustment traction. When the longitudinal force in the shaft of the penis is gradually increased, there will be multiplication of tissue cell leading to the penile tissue expansion. Tissue is added gradually to larger and longer penis.

E.USING KELGEL'S EXERCISE

When you carry out kelgel exercise ,your muscles will be enhance with the act of squeezing the muscles of your penis it is refer to as you finish the pee flow. You will be wrong if your stomach worked out of muscles. The muscles can be squeeze on and off. To end it, use the same muscle and start the pee flow again.

You can carry it out for about eight to ten set then you can go for a little break between set and resume back with twenty or twenty five daily

E.   USING   JELQUING EXERCISE

In this exercise, your thumbs is wrap up and place your finger at around the base of your penis and properly squeeze and press down your penis head. The action mainly assists in the increase of blood flow via the penis mainly when the penis is stretch. This exercise can be carried out using both the left and right hand and this will effectively increase the flow of blood to the penis.

F.USING THE CIRCULAR ROTATION

This exercise almost looks the same with stretching exercise but it has clear difference. This is how it works;

- ❖ Your penis should be hold with one hand and stretched out

* Then you can now rotate the penis in one direction for twenty five seconds

* You will now have to rotate the penis in the other direction for another twenty five seconds.

CHAPTER THREE

2. USING PLAN DIET.

If you are a man and you are eagerly searching for the best diet plan that can make your penis bigger and larger. This penis enlargement is determined by what is called genetics. The specific foods you need for penis enlargement training are discussed here. This specific food we are going to discuss here if combine with exercise, the quick result of bigger and stronger penis will be accomplished.

Vasodialators are some of the food you need in this training process for penis enlargement since they can increase blood flow directly to your penis. The following foods are listed below for penis enlargement.

I.   Liver

II.   Tuna

III.   Milk

IV.   Salmon

V.   Eggs

VI.   Vegetable such as carrots, tomatoes and sweet potatoes and broccoli

To increase the size of your penis without experiencing pain and side effects. Here are the three additional foods to the diet plan

that you must use for

speedy results·

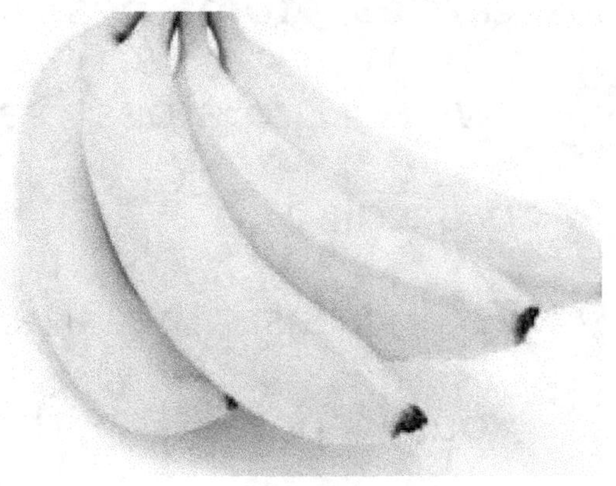

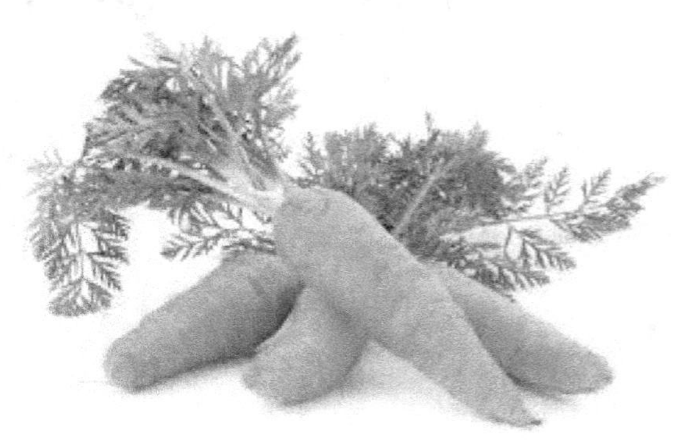

THE   USE   OF
PUMPKIN SEEDS

.

The use of pumpkin seeds as
a meal is very good and rich
in vitamin E. This vitamin E

helps to speed up blood to the penis

B.TAKING IN DARK CHOCOLATE

This is refer to as nutrient food because it helps in increasing sexual life and makes the blood flow to rise because it contains flavonol. This chocolate is loved by many persons because it is made from cocoa, it contain less sugar and also antioxidants.

Detoxifying your body can be achieved from this dark chocolate. A lot of calories are found in this dark chocolate to offer your body.

C.GINKGO BILOBA

This kind of food does not need to be forgotten for penis enlargement. If you are not use to this food try and add it to your meal and you will find it very interesting to have because it help circulate blood and help build your mind.

THE END

www.ingramcontent.com/pod-product-compliance
Lightning Source LLC
Chambersburg PA
CBHW051926250726
48659CB00002B/862